Got Bipolar?

An Insider's Guide to Managing Life Effectively

Alfredo Zotti

Loving Healing Press

Ann Arbor * Sydney

2nd Printing – April 2018

Library of Congress Cataloging-in-Publication Data

Names: Zotti, Alfredo, 1958- author.
Title: Got bipolar? : an insider's guide to managing life effectively / by
  Alfredo Zotti.
Description: Ann Arbor, MI : Loving Healing Press, [2017] | Includes
  bibliographical references and index.
Identifiers: LCCN 2017044718 (print) | LCCN 2017043563 (ebook) | ISBN
  9781615993642 (ePub, PDF, Kindle) | ISBN 9781615993628 (paperback
  : alk.paper) | ISBN 9781615993635 (hardcover : alk. paper) | ISBN
  9781615993659 (large print paperback : alk. paper) | ISBN
  9781615993642 (ebook : PDF, Kindle, ePub)
Subjects: LCSH: Manic-depressive illness--Treatment. | Manic-depressive
  persons--Psychology.
Classification: LCC RC516 (print) | LCC RC516 .Z684 2017 (ebook) |
DDC
  616.89/5--dc23
LC record available at https://lccn.loc.gov/2017044718

Distributed by: Ingram (USA/CAN/AU), Bertram's Books (UK, EU).

Published by:
Loving Healing Press
5145 Pontiac Trail
Ann Arbor, MI 48105

www.LHPress.com
info@LHPress.com

Table of Contents

Introduction

This book is about how to recover from bipolar disorder, or at least how to attempt to recover from it. The use of Emotional Regulation, Method Acting, Empathy Development, and Relaxation, which can be used to learn new skills that can help sufferers to recover, is covered briefly so you, the reader and sufferer, will need to do further research in order to get the best out of this book. The book will emphasize the right knowledge and skills the sufferer needs to develop. Because of the complexities of these issues, this book is just a guide, so the person needs to develop his or her own methods, based on this book's recommendations, in order to succeed.

Bipolar disorder is a serious condition that, as I have argued in previous books, and particularly in *Alfredo's Journey: An Artist's Creative Life with Bipolar Disorder* (Zotti, 2014), can interfere with the total health of the sufferer, making life very difficult. In the more severe cases, it can lead to suicide and cause much pain and discomfort not only to the person who suffers from it but for family members and friends.

Many people have learned how to cope with bipolar disorder and function reasonably well. They are said to have *recovered* from the disorder. Recovery does not mean cure; it simply means the person can function despite the symptoms and moods and is able to work toward a better life. In this sense, if you are someone who walks toward hope and has some positive thoughts, then this book is for you. If you are someone who lives in hopelessness and feels bipolar is a curse and that nothing will help, then it is doubtful anything will help until you break away from this damaging mindset.

Hope is not all that is needed. As you read this book, you will get to know the main ingredients necessary to recovery. Things like knowledge, good nutrition, good habits, adequate sleep, the right people around you (support group), and the right mental health professionals for you. You will realize that in order to walk toward recovery, you will need a support team of professionals and friends who will help, support, and understand you. If you are surrounded by people who make you feel bad, who drain your mind of all positivity, then it is unlikely you will be able to recover. The quality of your environment, both physical and social, is extremely important for good mental health.

In addition to these important factors, there are also strategies that can help you get on the road to recovery. One strategy I will mention here is that aspects and mechanisms of the acting profession can be used to help people who suffer with a mental disorder. It is not suggested that sufferers pick up acting as a profession because, as is commonly known, acting is a stressful job. For example, O'Neill (2015) argues that the demands of acting as a career are causing mental ill health for many struggling actors. We have all read something about the price of celebrity for actors who become famous.

What we are interested in is how Method Acting and Emotional Regulation can be useful in acquiring skills that help sufferers cope with mental ill health, symptoms such as depression and anxiety.

One of the most obvious benefits of acting is, as my friend Judy Wright puts it: "When performing, one dissociates from personal issues and focuses on telling a story. Maybe focusing outside ourselves makes it easier to regulate emotions."

I tend to agree with Judy that performing on stage can help us focus outside ourselves, making it easier for us to regulate emotions. However, this is easier said than done, particularly for people who have no access to a stage or to acting classes. Never fear—that is the reason for this book: to inform the reader what can be done to acquire an actor's skills. Just how would someone go about using acting skills to get out of debilitating depression?

Imagine you are in bed, unable to move due to severe depression. How can you help yourself? If you become high due to elevated moods, how can you help yourself? You are happy, the world is your oyster, and it is difficult to realize you are high and need to do something to calm yourself down. What to do?

Suggestions in this book will tell you to rely on others to understand your emotional and mental state. Listen to others and particularly those who are close and know you well. Ask a person you truly trust and who loves you to help you monitor your symptoms and moods, particularly if you happen to develop distorted thinking. A close person can be like a mirror for your emotions and moods and can really help you stay reasonably well. That person will gladly help you, and it is important you listen to and grow with him or her. This person might be your sister, brother, or mother. Ask the person to help you.

It is not just one thing that has to go right for someone to cope reasonably well, but a number of things. This means that coping reasonably well will depend on a balance between the right social environment, right opportunities, resilience of the person, and level of education, which has an impact on the person's psyche. We now begin to understand that the person has to work diligently to make all of this happen because our thoughts can impact our future and our life. We are not only what we eat but also our own thoughts. We are what we think we are, and what happens to us has a lot to do with what we think will happen to us.

What this book will show is that our ideology on mental disorders is very problematic. Today, it is clear for many enlightened mental health professionals that the mind's problems are not diseases. This is for two reasons: first, in the majority of cases of mental disorder, no specific physical causes can be identified; second, the problem has often to do with past traumas and the person's psyche (CDC, 2016; Read, Shannon, Douse, McCusker, Feeney, Barrett, Mullholland, 2011). The child is trapped in the adult body, unable to move on due to the trauma. Emotional growth is arrested or stumped. The trauma must be identified and worked upon for real improvement to show. My approach in this book can potentially help many sufferers with bipolar disorder.

In my many email communications with mental health professionals, I have frequently been told that people often take too much medication and do little or no therapy. If people go regularly to therapy and develop strategies to cope better, then they can reduce the amount of medication. Given that Post-

Traumatic Stress Disorder (PTSD) is present in the majority of cases of mental disorders, some say up to 85 percent, it is important to consider this advice from the more aware professionals.

It is also widely known, among the better and more educated mental health professionals, that the biopsychosocial model of any mental disorder is the right approach. This means a complete investigation and assessment of biological, psychological, and social factors that affect the person's wellbeing. Unfortunately, even in Australia, there is the tendency among the less skilled mental health professionals to see the problem as a purely biological one. But here is the problem that is very well-known among skilled mental health professionals:

> Conventional psychiatry is plagued by a confusion that lies at the very center of the conceptual problem of all modern, scientific medicine. Instead of asking why a mental illness occurs, medical researchers try to understand the biological mechanisms through which the illness operates. These mechanisms, rather than true origins, are seen as the causes of the illness. Accordingly, most current psychiatric treatments are limited to suppressing symptoms with psychoactive drugs. Although they have been successful in doing so, this approach has not helped psychiatrists to understand mental illness any better, nor has it allowed their patients to solve the underlying problems. (R.D. Laing in Capra, 1988)

Common sense is important. Believe it or not, even some doctors and mental health professionals lack common sense when it comes to mental disorders. For example, what is the use of medicating a woman who is constantly beaten by her partner? It is clear she needs to escape domestic violence if her condition is to improve. No medication available today will compensate for the trauma she endures every day.

A doctor, or other mental health professional, should always ask what the likely social and environmental problems may be before jumping to medication. Medication, in unfavorable cases, can be more harmful than good: for example, an overdose that leads to suicide or side effects, or addiction to drugs (Reznik, 2006).

Because of all of the above reasons, my suggestion is never to stop asking for help, any help, be it financial or otherwise. There is nothing wrong with asking for help, and one way to ensure we become used to seeking the right help is to write to specific organizations that can help us like Lifeline or SANE. Writing or speaking to such organizations will let them know what we need and will often lead to some help. Even the act of speaking to someone about one's problems is enough to make a huge difference, particularly when a sufferer is contemplating suicide.

This book is about solving underlying problems and helping the person to recover. To conclude this introduction, if you suffer with bipolar and want to recover, there is always a need to attend to the psychological (what is in your mind, how you see the problems, and how you respond to life's problems), social (the people around you—are they helpful to you? Are they supportive?), and biological (in terms of finding the right medication that will help you).

Chapter 1 - Ingredients Important for Recovery

Knowledge of Bipolar Disorder

At the top of the recipe, we put "knowledge of the disorder." What is bipolar disorder and what causes it? These are the million-dollar questions to which professionals and writers have provided different answers, and in this sense, we have different perspectives.

Basically, there are those who feel that "there is only a brain" and the brain malfunctions in bipolar disorder. The malfunction is permanent and the only solution for this defect is medication first and therapy second. This is not my view.

Then there are those who propose that there is a mind, not just a brain. Medication is a crutch that is good at the beginning, and it is certainly good for the more severe types of bipolar, and therapy is always needed for us to learn coping mechanisms and simply to talk about our problems with a professional, friend, or family member. However, for true recovery, the sufferer has to do a lot of work, a lot of the right work. In this sense, I am on the side of those who propose that, while everything is in the brain, there are also stories and worldviews that matter a lot because stories and worldviews can influence our thinking or the brain's functioning. Stories and worldviews take on a life of their own, even though they are abstract things, and we absorb these stories and worldviews with our brain.

While I agree that life is a product of brain functions, it is also true that the brain creates worldviews and stories. Indeed, stories are part of our life. We make sense of our life based on the story we are told, the stories we tell others, and the stories we tell ourselves. These stories are based on specific knowledge we acquire. These stories make a tremendous difference in how we see our disorder, how we cope with it, and whether we are to recover.

Yes, brain functions are important, but worldviews and the story we use to understand the world are equally important. In this sense, there is not just a brain but a mind that comprises both brain and worldviews or stories. It is much like hardware and software in the computer world. The brain is the hardware and the worldviews and stories are the software. However, the brain is not exactly like computer hardware because, unlike computer hardware, it can re-adjust itself and even heal itself. Norman Doidge explains this in his famous book *The Brain That Changes Itself* (2007). In this sense, the brain is plastic, and even when its hardware is broken, other parts of the brain can take over new functions. The brain is miraculous, and that is why recovery is possible. And that is also why it is important to use the best software that can help the hardware readjust itself. This perspective is the one I like best.

Helpful Books

Of course, a lot more knowledge exists about bipolar disorder than I can give you in this small volume, so you will need to read as much as you can to acquire the knowledge that can help you recover. The books that have helped my wife and me, and that I suggest you read, are only four to start with, but they are important for recovery. These are:

Capra, F. (1989). *Uncommon wisdom: conversations with remarkable people*. Flamingo: Hammersmith, London.

Corry, A., Tubridy, A. (2001). *Going MAD? Understanding mental illness*. Newleaf: Dublin.

Harris, Thomas A. (1973). *I'm OK—You're OK*. Pan Books: London, Sydney, Auckland.

Zotti, A. (2014). *Alfredo's journey: An artist's creative life with bipolar disorder*. Modern History Press: Ann Arbor, MI.

You can read short passages from these books, and I suggest that you read them over and over so you can really grasp what is said. I have read them many times and continue to read them to this day. Think about what you read and see how it relates to your bipolar disorder. These books have helped me tremendously, and I would not have been able to recover without them. You can add to your personal collection of helpful books and help your knowledge—the right knowledge—to grow. These books will provide the foundations for you to build upon. They agree with my perspective that the mind is made up of hardware and software, but, unlike conventional hardware, the brain can heal itself because it is plastic. Given that traumatic experiences are often the root cause of many mental disorders, hope and recovery are real.

Nutrition

What should you eat? This is an interesting question. Before I suggest what to eat it is important to understand that food is better than medication for us. Indeed, certain foods contain ingredients that can help our depression and our elevated moods. Depending on how we feel, we have to learn to use the right foods. For example, you should not drink coffee when you are experiencing elevated moods. No caffeine, no nicotine and no alcohol. Alcohol is a depressant. It may make you feel a bit better while you are drinking and inebriated but this is followed by deep and dangerous depression that can lead to suicidal ideation.

When it comes to nutrition, I could give you a very long list about what to eat and what not to eat, but the thing is that the best way to put together the kind of nutrition that will help you is by doing research and trying to match the food that is good with the food that you tolerate or like. We are all different. What is important to know, however, is that food is medicine because that is where medicines partly come from: plants and food. Antioxidants, for example, prevent cell damage while smart carbohydrates can have a calming effect. vitamin D, selenium-rich foods and omega-3 fatty acids are all good for your bipolar, and will help tremendously. Fruits, vegetables, nuts, all fresh foods will help you feel better and cope better with your bipolar disorder. It is important to have some written material on good nutrition and consult a health professional about your choices of food, food that you think that will help your mental disorder. I cannot stress enough how important it is to eat good nutritious food and to stay away from recreational drugs, tobacco and alcohol.

Love Yourself

Loving yourself does not equate to being selfish or vain. It means to study yourself carefully and be able to understand yourself and your place in the universe.

One of the most important things to learn is that from suffering comes wisdom and the ability to find peace. If you are suffering, whether it is due to depression or anything else, it is important to know that that suffering is not in vain, but is there for a reason. It is the seed from which resilience can grow, if you learn to see the situation from the right perspective. This is a concept that the Polish psychiatrist Kazmierz Dabrowski had written extensively about after having survived two world wars and seen many atrocities. There is a thesis online, written by Battaglia (2002) about his life and I feel that you will benefit from reading it[1].

There are many other expressions of this important idea, which I agree with. Friedrich Nietzsche: "What doesn't kill you makes you stronger."[2]

A lot of research has also been done on post-traumatic growth. Once we understand this concept, it is not difficult to entertain the idea that it is important to be willing to feel pain and understand its origins. It is important to embrace our feelings and emotions rather than to run away from then, hide them in our subconscious, or dismiss them altogether. Our emotions and feelings are important, so we need to understand them and their causation. It is good to breathe in a few minutes in our day and learn to get in touch with our feelings and emotions, to accept them, study them, and learn how not to suffer as much next time around. It is vital not to run away from our emotions and feelings and not to make others responsible for how we feel. No one can make us feel bad if we don't want to let them. Only we can make ourselves feel bad about something.

It is important to study and learn as much as possible about yourself and psychology so you can learn how to protect yourself from pain, how to cope with difficult situations, and how to

---

[1] https://theses.lib.vt.edu/theses/available/etd-04082002-204054/unrestricted/Dissertation.pdf

[2] http://www.dailymail.co.uk/sciencetech/article-2075908/So-Nietzsche-WAS-right-What-doesnt-kill-makes-stronger-scientists-find.html

enjoy what is good or can be good in your life. We all have a higher self inside of us, a self that instinctively knows how to help ourselves. It is important to get in touch with this higher self and learn how to be in harmony with the Universe's energy. A great reminder of this is the "Desiderata Letter" written by Max Ehermann in 1927. I think it is helpful to read this letter over and over to get its important message (see Appendix A).

False Beliefs & Distorted Thinking

Learn as much as possible about your false beliefs and distorted thinking. These are real enemies that prevent wellbeing and your ability to cope and develop resilience. However, the recovery process is a long one, with many relapses. One thing to know is that after failing a few times, you will be able to recover well if you really want to.

What is distorted thinking? Because most people with bipolar disorder have experienced trauma during childhood, their thinking has the danger of being stuck in a childish pattern when trauma is triggered. We respond to events-now in a way that may have been appropriate for events-back-then. This is distorted thinking. We may see enemies where there are none; we may misinterpret people's true intentions, and we may see enemies, failure, and disaster everywhere we look. This is not always so, but often our distorted thinking makes us perceive things in this negative way. Of course, people have violated our trust in the past, which is why we are so suspicious that our thinking sometimes becomes distorted. It is important not to trust yourself completely when making decisions and judgments but to learn to wait, consult people who can advise you, and act only when you have considered the situation fully and when you have the advice of experienced people who can help you. This alone will avoid much pain in your life. In an email exchange, Dr. Robert Rich wrote:

> Part of the reason for my healing was when I realized that my opinion of myself was the internalization of my stepfather's opinion of me as a child. I kept abusing myself by believing his untruths about me. So, when a thought of self-hate came, I refused to buy into it. Instead, I examined it in the light of the evidence, which was

things like my achievements, the opinions of people around me, how others responded to the same situation, etc.

The higher self in you knows when you are doing well, when your intentions are good, and when you productively work toward contributing to the universe's energy. Learn to get in touch with this higher self, and when you do a good thing, pat yourself on the back and be proud of yourself. If you fail, you should never bash yourself up, but forgive yourself and tell yourself that you will do much better next time, that you will do your best to change to avoid the same problem again. Treat every failure as a learning opportunity, which it is until you will eventually not fail anymore.

Speak to your feelings and emotions, learn about them, and evaluate your actions. Don't run away from the problems and how you feel about them. Sure, you will probably suffer more in the short term, but in the long term, you will learn to cope better and develop resilience. Don't be afraid to suffer; get used to it, provided that the suffering is natural and not self-inflicted. We can learn a lot from suffering. In fact, that is what makes us stronger people.

Loving yourself in this way will improve everything in your life; it will make you a much better person and open up new pathways for you to succeed in anything you do.

It is not as simple as reading this book. You will have to work really hard at it, but at least this book provides some ideas about how to go about learning to love yourself. It does not matter if you have faults, because all humans do, and sometimes faults or defects can become valuable if seen from novel perspectives. Consider the parable of "The Cracked Pot" (see Appendix A). Read it and you will understand why we are all special no matter what affliction, disabilities, or defects we may have. There is always a way for us to change and become better people, able to love ourselves and others.

Chapter 2 - Recovery

What Matters: Toward Recovery

When it comes to recovery, what matters is not how mild or severe our mental disorder is, but how we travel inside: Are we traveling toward recovery? Or are we traveling toward despair?

In my experience, as a volunteer helper for many people online, most people travel toward hopelessness and despair because they have been convinced there is no hope for their condition. This is simply wrong because there is plenty of hope for any condition, no matter how severe.

Wellbeing is achievable, so people with psychiatric disorders must become active when it comes to their behavior and symptoms and the related management of them. People become active participants in the choices, self-determination, and personal responsibilities that enable them to embark on the road toward recovery, and the expertise of consumers is acknowledged and valued.

Fighting Stigma and Myths

Stigma and myths are a barrier to these achievements, but it is important for all people to remember that stigma and myths are just that—myths, which are far removed from the truth. People with mental disorders are said to be dangerous, irresponsible, dependent, and incompetent. While all people can be these things, mental disorder or not, the reality is that the majority of people with mental disorders are not dangerous, are not irresponsible, and are not dependent or incompetent. They are just experiencing problems that often have to do with an unhealthy integration with the social and physical environment.

For people to be well integrated with their social and physical environment, it is necessary to stay connected with things like history, education, friends, work, politics, hopes, dreams, beliefs, values, and everything that is important in a person's life. But what happens for people with mental disorders is that because they become alienated, due to stigma and myths around mental disorders. They often lose friends; become alienated from their history; distance themselves from education (a system that unfortunately is often riddled with stigma); develop problems with family members and, therefore, distance themselves from family; lose interest in politics; and lose the ability to dream and hope for social norms and society. It is important for the sufferers to be aware of these problems and to begin to work either with a person of trust who understands about mental disorders, or, ideally, with a therapist toward reestablishing a connection with these things so healthy relationships can be restored. *But how?*

The Negative Ideology of Mental Disorders

For one thing, it is important to become aware of the negative ideology of mental disorders and its impact on the person. The negative ideology has a negative impact on self-concept, efficacy, hopes and dreams, emotions, major social roles, and engagement with the helping systems. The person experiences loss of sense of self, loss of connectedness, guilt, shame, isolation, loss of power, loss of valued role, and finally, loss of hope (Spaniol & Khohler, 1999; Rosnik et. al., 1999).

It becomes evident that a person with a mental disorder, when confronted with these problems and this ideology, is forced to cope with the catastrophe of mental disorder and multiple and recurring traumas—the trauma from the mental disorder and the trauma from how he or she is treated in society. Professionals often have negative attitudes influenced largely by a system of seeing mental illness as an end in itself rather than a problem that has an origin that can be attended and worked upon. And finally, the person is confronted with the incompetence of professionals who lack the appropriate skills and understanding they should have.

In contrast to this situation, we can embrace the new paradigm according to which, as McGruder writes (2001)

> The social power to define and categorize another person's experience is not a power to be ignored...in order

to support persons who are trying to recover, we must attend to the fullness of their experiences, and not be distracted by their medical diagnosis.

The science of psychiatric diagnosis and treatment is neither objective, nor neutral nor value free. Rather, it is a social process open to bias and influenced by the larger social, political and cultural milieu.

According to this new paradigm of mental disorders, the right attitude toward recovery is manifested by, as Clay (1990, p. 232) argues, a specific attitude:

> The person most likely to get well—to become empowered—is the person who feels free to question, to accept or reject treatment, and to communicate with and care for people who are caring for her or him....
>
> Ultimately, patient empowerment is a matter of self determination; it occurs when a patient freely chooses his or her own path to recovery and wellbeing. It is the job of the mental health services to provide an environment of personal respect, material support, and social justice that encourage the individual person in this process.

Barriers to Recovery

So what prevents sufferers from recovery? I have already touched on this elsewhere, but for the sake of clarity and efficiency, here are some important points:

- The greatest obstacle to one's recovery is simply that most sufferers think they cannot recover. This, of course, is totally wrong; it is a distorted way of perceiving something that is not true.

- That one cannot control moods and symptoms. This again is false. For example, I have succeeded at this. My wife has also been able to control her moods and symptoms, and so have hundreds of sufferers I have tried to help online.

- It is not just one factor that is important in controlling moods and symptoms but many: therapy is always necessary no matter what because, among other things, it is not easy to cope with a mental disorder whatever its origins may be, so that discussing one's struggles always helps. Medication can help, especially in the initial stages; use the minimum amount possible that is effective. But medication only buys time till the sufferer gains skills to help him- or herself, and in this sense, it requires hard work. At one stage, for recovery, the hard work must be done.

- Avoiding recreational drugs, alcohol, cigarettes, and even coffee is helpful. If you must use these substances, then use the minimal amount possible. These substances will make your mental disorder worse. Even caffeine can be dangerous for someone experiencing elevated moods.

- Good nutrition and exercise are vital for staying reasonably well.

- It is also necessary to create for oneself a reasonably stress-free life. One cannot expect, for example, to live in a domestic violence situation and be able to work toward recovery. This is not going to happen. One must first remove the problem, in this case the domestic violence, and them attempt to work toward recovery.

- Full resilience can be developed with the help of knowledge and books. It is important to develop a certain critical con-sciousness in which we start to study ourselves, our thinking, and our habits, and to question them in a constructive manner. Positive self-criticism is vital in the recovery process.

- It is vitally important to work with a therapist and try to ascertain whether the mental disorder originates from a traumatic experience. Research tells us that most mental disorders originate in childhood or from childhood traumas. Finding the trauma and working on it can be wonderfully therapeutic, but also stressful and difficult. Still, it's worth it for those who are courageous. Indeed, if PTSD (Post Traumatic Stress Disorder) is present, then it is necessary to work on it for any recovery to be possible.

- Learn a bit about the mind and particularly read about abnormal psychology.

- Create your own support group of mental health profes-sionals who are understanding; of friends who can support you; of family members who can help you and understand. Eliminate toxic people who are prejudiced toward you. Don't build up resentment or animosity toward people. Simply avoid those who are prejudiced and find comfort in those who understand and help you. Many good people are out there.

- Become aware that mental disorders distort our thinking. To understand and pinpoint the distorted thought, it is necessary to be honest with a person of trust or a therapist and find the courage to open up and observe the distorted thinking.

- Learn to let emotions out. Crying can also be very therapeutic; it cleanses the soul. Even tough men can cry, and indeed, they should sometimes to free the bottled-up emotions.

- Find an activity you like and make it your hobby. Creative activities are particularly beneficial because they help us get caught up in the moment, focusing on the task at hand and forgetting our problems. This gives our brain a chance to recharge and break the constant rumination that is often part of the depressive cycle.

- Accept your disorder as a part of you and turn it into something positive. For example, depression gives rise to my creativity when it lifts. I know it does not last forever but is only a temporary setback. That is how, in my mind, I turn a negative into a positive.

If you follow what I said here, and you practice it regularly, you will be well on your way to recovery. Recovery does not mean to be cured of moods and symptoms, but simply that we learn to live with these defects and make the best of our life learning to cope with them, even turning them into strengths that can help us.

Finally, as the stoic philosopher Epictetus wrote, happiness and freedom begin with a clear understanding of one principle: Some things are within our control but many are not. Life is unpredictable, so we must accept what we can control and what we cannot. Acceptance is also the key to recovery.

Resilience

What is resilience when speaking of a mental disorder? It is what allows us to recover from traumas or adverse life experiences: to bounce back. We can be knocked down by life events and come back stronger than ever if we have adequate resilience. Alternatively, we can develop it with proper help. Cognitive Behavioral Therapy (CBT) can be useful for us if we desire to develop resilience. We may be overwhelmed by events like the loss of a loved one or being involved in a severe car accident, or we may cope. Such resilience can be developed. Let me give you an example from my past.

I used to have very little resilience; in fact, I was at the mercy of my moods, so when bipolar depression came, I was confined to my bed. I could not get up, nor did I have any intention of getting up. I was constantly ruminating, and my repeating thoughts made me feel worse and worse. They took up so much of my energy that I felt as if I couldn't even lift an arm. It was horrible—the most severe depression, the deepest black hole I have ever experienced—with no way out on the horizon. What to do?

It was not until I met Dr. Robert Rich and started to talk to sufferers online that it became clear to me that this rumination and that voice, which kept telling me how terrible the world was, how miserable life was, how hopeless my situation was, and that all I should do was stay in bed and not move till I finally died, was just a mirage my mind had created. The effect was real, the depression was certainly there, but the idea that there was no hope was not true. It was a mirage created by the mind, a mirage of hopelessness and doom.[3]

I soon began to fight against it. If the voice told me not to get up, I would do the best to get up, even if the pain was excruciating. It felt like my bones would break if I kept moving. But I persevered and got out of bed. After I did it once, with enormous difficulty, it became easier the second time. Soon, the depression would not hold me in bed all day, and I also learned how to cope with depression, how to continue to function while depressed. It was far from easy; it was painful and terribly hard. In fact, I think it was the most difficult thing I had to learn in life—to continue to live while depressed. But I did it and soon the depression lifted. Over the years, I learned how to ride the depression, knowing that eventually it would lift. The best way to deal with the monster called depression is to defy it.

---

[3] http://bobswriting.com/psych/firstaid.com

What has been happening for me over the years is that by talking to other people who understand bipolar disorder, and by creating a network of people who have been able to support me during difficult times, I have developed resilience. In other words—and this is the most important thing you will learn from this book—you need to create a support group for yourself, a support group that understands your bipolar disorder and can help. *But who?* you may ask. My wife had no family, and I was not in touch with mine for many years. We had no one to support us, but eventually, we created a network of mental health professionals who were sympathetic to our struggles: our doctor Cavanagh; our psychologist Paul Corcoran; and the friends I made online, even if I never met them in person, like my friends Judy Wright and Rosemary Martin. These people have supported me, and this supportive network is what has really helped me to develop resilience.

It is important to mention that I also gave my brain a break from the constant rumination. I did this by taking my mind off everything while playing music, writing poetry, painting and drawing, and writing academically. I did creative things, and that creativity gave my mind a chance to recharge to get away from the draining rumination. To ruminate all the time without stopping is a very bad thing to do; it just sucks all of the energy from you. It is extremely important to learn to engage in an activity that will help you become at one with what you are doing, and, therefore, escape the rumination, even if only for a few minutes. It is surprising to find that even a few minutes away from the rumination will give your mind a chance to recharge.

Steps for Successfully Coping

In summary, the following steps are important:

- **Learn to engage in an activity that will help you get away from the rumination** when depressed. Forget your problems and everything to do with your life for a while and have a hobby, no matter what it is—gardening, writing, painting, playing music, or any other activity that will help you take your mind off your problems and off the rumination. Rumination, or the act of ruminating, can become addictive and even comforting, or so we think. But it is really very destructive.

- **Don't be afraid to ask for help.** Find people who know you and your mental disorder and are able to support you. If you tell them how you feel, chances are they will help you learn how to cope. Not singly or immediately, but over time, you will find that their efforts were helpful. When you combine the help of many people, you find that this collective effort will help you to cope. It takes time, though; it does not happen overnight.

- **Create a network of people,** even online (for example join a self-help site where you can communicate with other sufferers for a while). This network should comprise some mental health professionals who can help you, some friends with the same affliction, or anyone willing to listen to and support you. A network is tremendously important because, let's face it, stigma is going to be out there in society, and you will find it time and time again in your life. However, it is absolutely important not to internalize it; understand that stigma and prejudice are not our problem; we don't have to be with people who are prejudiced, and we do not have to put up with it. We can simply move away and find supportive people who are not prejudiced. But, whatever we do, it is vital not to internalize stigma in the way many sufferers do.

- **Do not internalize stigma.** What do I mean by internalizing stigma? I internalize stigma when I believe I am faulty because I have this condition. It is when I am the person who stigmatizes me. When this happens, we can come to hate everything, even ourselves, and it is a destructive thing to do. Internalizing the world's problems is quite silly: we cannot eradicate racism; we cannot eradicate the negative sentiments people have against homosexuals or lesbians; we cannot expect all people to be nice.

The world is complex, and there is good and bad, but there is no need for us to listen to others' opinions. We have to learn to avoid negativity and people who are prejudiced against us. Life will never be perfect, but it can be good if we make it good. If we believe what these prejudiced people are saying, that is internalizing the problem. These people, however, are wrong because to have a mental illness is not only a problem; it can also be a blessing. There is always negative and positive in everything.

- **Remember thoughts are powerful**, so thinking negatively all the time will have a detrimental impact on every aspect of life. Thoughts create reality. Everything around us comes from someone's thoughts: the car we drive, the clothes we wear, the perfume we put on, the television, everything around us comes from thought. Thought can also impact our chances and opportunities. It's vital to learn to have some positive thoughts in our repertoire of thinking if we want to develop resilience.

- **Accept life** and understand that material things alone, without spiritual values in our life, lead to unhappiness. We do not need to be rich, to have a fast car, to have the best clothes and the best shoes to be happy, despite what the media wants us to believe. We need to become better people, and in order to achieve this, we need to develop patience, to learn how to be content with what we have, as opposed to wanting what we can't have immediately.

  Acceptance and delaying gratification are part of wisdom, and it is important to develop some wisdom in life. Happiness is not based just on what material possessions we have or what we can show others to prove we are affluent. Our consumer society wants us to believe that material things are a symbol of who we are, but this could not be further from the truth. Even very rich and famous people are unhappy.

- **Find the right books to read**, or the right literature to read online. Books on meditation and relaxation, and especially audio books on relaxation can also be very helpful.

- **Learn to forgive yourself.** This is important because, let's face it, we are going to make mistakes time and time again. If we have bipolar disorder, and we have not developed the right resilience and knowledge, chances are that we are programmed for negativity. Life, under the cloud of a negative mind, can only be problematic. When we make mistakes, we need to realize they also result from our condition, our distorted thinking, and our misperceptions and exaggerations. Albert Einstein is credited with saying, "The person who never made a mistake never tried anything new."

Our perception can be distorted at times, or in some situations, and this is understandable given that our past is, in many bipolar cases, traumatic This will have led us to lose trust in people. According to statistics, 85 percent of people with bipolar have experienced documented trauma in their childhoods. The right people will understand and forgive us. The wrong people won't be able to, but then we don't really need the wrong people in our lives, if we can help it.

If we really have to deal with the wrong people, for example, if we have a non-understanding boss at work, then we may have to find strategies around that or, alternatively, if it is not possible to use strategies with some people, then we need to get those people out of our lives. Sometimes, leaving a job that makes us unwell may be necessary for our own state of mind, for our own health.

- **Study and read as much as possible about bipolar disorder and talk to people who suffer with the same disorder.** You need to become your own therapist; you need to be able to discuss your problems and find other people who may be facing the same dilemmas you face.

To recapitulate this chapter, here is what you need to do, in point form. Please memorize this and explore the possibilities:

- Engage in helpful and creative activities.
- Learn to ask for help from the right people.
- Create a network of supporting people.
- Understand your thoughts and how powerful they are.
- Accept life with all its problems and faults. Life is not perfect and neither are people.
- Find the right literature that will help you. (I will suggest many books in a separate chapter).
- Learn to forgive yourself and try to do better next time.
- Study as much as possible, especially humanities subjects like anthropology, sociology, history, psychology, or philosophy. Knowledge is necessary for

people with bipolar disorder. The more we know, the better we can cope.

"Social Support"

As Rufus May argues (2007):

> Recovery requires other people to believe in and stand by the person. Other people/opportunities play an important part in enabling the person to make this recovery journey.

Social support is vital. Indeed, a social network of supporting people can truly help the person to recover. This supporting network should be made of some mental health professionals such as your doctor, your therapist, or a social worker; supportive friends; supportive family members; supportive colleagues; or any person who knows you fairly well and is supportive and understanding of your mental disorder.

Chapter 3 - Method Acting and Emotional Regulation

Method Acting

Since the 1930s, method acting has evolved through experimentation, but the main principles remain the same. The aim is to create a lifelike, credible character, to escape the pitfalls of simple impersonation, and to *become* the character. In a way, method acting is not really acting as such, but the personification of a character. Method acting requires certain skills that are acquired only when the actor has a vast knowledge of the method, of human nature, and of emotional regulation.

It is far from easy to be able to practice method acting because of its emotional intensity and the bravery required. When we use method acting, we are attempting to create a performance that is emotionally truthful, and we need to believe in the character we are playing; we become the character. This can have its dangers, but as we apply it here, namely to create a character that is fairly happy and content with his or her life, it can only lead to positive outcomes.

After you finish reading this book and gain the relevant knowledge on bipolar disorder, you may wish to try these steps:

- Learn as much as possible about Stanislavsky's Method of Acting.

- Write yourself a script about a character that is positive, happy, and content in his or her life (no matter how problematic your own life may be).

- Create a character that will motivate and interest you enough to want to continue playing that character.

- Practice and practice the character until it becomes second nature to play him or her. In all probability, if you do succeed in playing this character, your life will change for the better just as my life has changed. Our mental activity can also produce reality and thus impact our lives.

Simply stated, the argument here presented is that aspects and mechanisms of the acting profession can be used to help people who suffer with a mental disorder. It is not suggested that sufferers pick up acting as a profession because, as is commonly known, acting is a stressful job. For example, O'Neill (2015) argues that the demands of acting, as a career, are causing mental health issues for many struggling actors. On the other hand, we have all read something about the price of celebrity for actors who become famous.

Acting as a Coping Mechanism

What we are interested in is how subjects like method acting and emotional regulation can be useful in helping sufferers acquire skills that help them cope with mental health issues such as depression and anxiety.

One of the most obvious benefits of acting is, as my friend Judy Wright puts it:

> "When performing, one dissociates from personal issues and focuses on telling a story. Maybe focusing outside ourselves makes it easier to regulate emotions."

I tend to agree with Judy that performing on stage can help us focus outside ourselves, thereby making it easy for us to regulate emotions. However, this is easier said than done, particularly for people who have no access to a stage or to acting classes. Never fear. The whole reason for this book is to inform the reader about what can be done to acquire some acting skills. Just how would a person go about using acting skills to get out of a debilitating depression? Perhaps the person is in bed, unable to move due to severe depression. How can that person help him- or herself?

When one is depressed, one ruminates: that is, a person keeps thinking about negative thoughts that go round and round in one's mind, in circle, indefinitely. Breaking the cycle of the rumination is extremely difficult. Some argue that it is the rumination that causes depression, while others say a biological brain defect causes the rumination. Both may be right, but ultimately, this is a chicken-or-the-egg kind of question.

In my opinion, both as a sufferer of bipolar 2 and as a full-time caregiver to my wife who suffers from bipolar 1, acting skills can help. The actor has to, by necessity, put him- or herself in another character's shoes, whether it be a real character or a fictitious one. In order to do so, the actor has to take on the characteristics of a new personality. In other words, the actor has to be able to store and retrieve a variety of emotions, feelings, and states of mind that go with the character.

If there is need to play a depressed person, the actor will do it; if there is need to assume the character of an extremely happy person, the actor will do it; and this is regardless of how he or she really feels inside. Sure, an actor can try to prepare, to have a very relaxing and peaceful time days before performing, but in the end, life goes on, and even if actors experience problems in their lives, the show must go on. Indeed, the show *must* go on, and this is the key.

What if a sufferer were to learn how to stop ruminating at once, after much practice—to go in front of the mirror and pretend that he or she is happy, and even smile. *I am going to be OK today*, she or he tells the mirror. *I am going to be a different character today, one full of hope and zest for life regardless of whether inside I feel like I am dying. I am going to act to feel better.*

Is this possible? If you were to ask my wife and me, we would say yes, it is perfectly possible because we do it often. Indeed, my wife suffered from terrible depression and often needed hospitalization. But with hard work, we have been able to develop skills, similar to those used by the actor, so we can break the rumination, even if for a short while. This break is enough for the brain to recharge, to escape the constant worries and rumination that are a real drain on energies, on the nervous system, and on personality. In this way, the person gets a break from the rumination, which makes all of the difference.

Emotional Regulation

Emotional regulation is a complex area. Although I can write just a few words in the space of this short booklet, it is important for you to do further research.

Actors are basically interested in learning to control emotional reactions by monitoring, evaluating, and modifying emotions. To give an example, suppressing emotional reactions is not good for our health. With PTSD, people hide their emotions by necessity, automatically, because a response of the mind, confronted by overwhelming events such as the death of a loved one, rape, or war—to name a few—are blocked by the mind so that no damage can be inflicted on the psyche or the self. However, these bottled-up emotions, feelings, and memories will need to come out sooner or later if the people are to recover from their traumatic experiences.

How do actors respond to a particular situation? How do they modulate or control their emotions? Your task in this exercise is to practice how to regulate and modify your emotions so you can play the character of a reasonably happy and content person, even if you are really hurting inside. The show must go on after all. This is the emotional intensity and courage that a good actor develops—the courage to try something new, to experience new emotions and feelings. The courage to abandon one's old character even if for a few hours or minutes. Read about this topic and learn as much as possible about it.

Life as a Recovering Actor

Who and what is a recovering actor? In my opinion, a recovering actor is someone who suffers with a mental disorder and attempts to use an aspect of an acting career to recover from his or her mental disorder. In other words, if we feel extremely depressed, we have to act to look happy. Is this even possible? Yes, it is very possible but not easy. It takes enormous determination, practice, and courage.

This does not mean a person suffering from depression or anxiety should just snap out of it. It simply means that we can learn to function despite the symptoms. I do it often, as does my wife and many of my friends. We continue to function despite the symptoms that, had we not developed strategies and coping skills, would be totally debilitating.

As recovering actors, we must learn to do research about things that are important to our lives. We must learn as much as possible about our mental disorder; we must communicate with other sufferers and compare their suffering to our own to see differences and similarities; we must read books that speak of recovery and hope and tell us it is possible to find happiness no matter what is wrong with us—that every single human being on Earth has some sort of disorder or disability. No one is perfect, and indeed, life is not perfect.

We are special actors, not theater actors, who work to improve our own lives. But there are similarities, and some methods are the same. Accordingly, it is very helpful to read as much as possible about method acting. Imagine you are an actor. You happen to feel depressed, anxious, tired or whatever. How can you function despite your symptoms? Actors do it often, for no matter how they feel, the show must go on. I have a few friends who are actors. One day I was communicating with a well-known actor who also suffers with bipolar disorder. He said (I'm paraphrasing to hide the actor's identity):

> Sometimes, it is possible to postpone filming, if an actor does not feel well, but sometimes, it is just not possible due to time limitations and budget. In my last film, I was extremely depressed. I had to play the part of a child molester, and that was extremely difficult for me because I love children. I was extremely depressed, but I went in front of my bathroom mirror and forced myself to smile. Inside, I felt like I was dying, that the world would end tomorrow. But you know, soon after the first forced smile, I started to feel better. It was incredible how just the attempt to do something helpful makes us immediately feel better. Yet when you are closed up in your depression, you feel nothing can help. It is true to say that depression is a great liar, a monster that wants you to believe nothing will help and your life is over. But it is not true.

What is important for us, at this stage, is to understand how we can empower ourselves and how we can get on the road to recovery. In order to play our character, we need knowledge. We need to understand that our effort here is to learn to cope and function well with our mental disorder, and to do this, we can begin with social and environmental issues and then move to the personal.

The Reality of Hope

It is extremely important to understand that what matters toward recovery is not how severe our mental disorder is, but how we travel in our mind: Are we traveling toward hope and the effort to improve our life? Or are we traveling toward hopelessness and despair? If we look around us, it is easy to entertain the idea that most people with a mental disorder today travel toward hopelessness and despair, and the reason for this is our problematic social world and how mental disorders are seen from a very wrong perspective. Rather than ask ourselves, "What caused the depression or the anxiety, or whatever other mental disorder?" we rush to look at the symptoms and treat them as an illness, a malfunction of the brain.

Evidence shows (Felitti, 1998) that most people suffering from mental disorders have experienced childhood trauma. This is the root cause of the problem. This requires therapy or the ability to discuss one's problems with a therapist or at least someone with knowledge who is willing to listen. We also need the necessary acquisition of knowledge. What we are here doing for recovery is changing the software to a level where we can function. And by changing our mental software, we will slowly change the hardware of our brain. Knowledge is essential for recovery, and we need to become knowledgeable actors, because for recovery, we first need to act our way out of the pit of despair. For this to happen, we must want to walk toward recovery and out of despair.

The Prognosis of Doom must be replaced with the Reality of Hope. The main message is that we can recover; we can get better. This does not mean we will stop experiencing symptoms, but it does mean we can learn how to cope with them and even gain positive outcomes from the suffering. Is this possible? Of course it is; my wife and I are living prove that this is possible. Many others would say the same.

Become an Active Participant

People with mental disorders are no longer passive recipients of symptoms and behavioral interventions given by professionals who accept whatever treatment is given to them. We need to become active in our recovery, become educated about medication, about therapy, about our particular disorder, and work with our therapist toward recovery. This is the way forward.

We need to learn to make the right choices, with the advice of experienced people who work with us. We need to become responsible for our lives. We need to promote a world where sufferers with mental disorders are recognized as valuable members of society.

In order to do this, we must understand that many people usually see those of us with mental disorders as dangerous, incompetent, dependent on others, and irresponsible. This could not be further from the truth and, as recovering actors, we must begin to act in such a way that we can dispel these myths. For a healthy integration with our society, we need to be in sync with our hopes, values, and beliefs; we need to attempt to create a supportive environment with people who can support us and understand us; we need to develop a certain spiritual under-standing of life, not necessarily religious but one based on the idea that everything is connected in the Universe by an invisible energy, perhaps collective consciousness. Work, education, politics, our past, our friends, and everything that is part of life is important; we need to synchronize ourselves with these social institutions so we can be part of society. What prevents us from doing this is the negative impact that the main ideology on mental illness has on us. But we can act our way out of this damaging ideology.

The Importance of Hobbies

Having a hobby is extremely important because when we engage in an activity we like—be it painting with colors, writing poetry, collecting stamps, working with plants and keeping a garden, or whatever activity makes us happy—we forget about our problems and, most importantly, we stop ruminating. This gives our brain a chance to refresh itself to recover from the constant drains of the worries and the negative circular thinking that is part of our bipolar disorder.

I could write a lot about this topic, but the truth is that I have already written extensively about it in: Pearson, C., Mann, S., Zotti, A., (2016) *Art Therapy and the Creative Process: a critical approach*. Loving Healing Press, Ann Arbor. I think would be really good for you to read. If you cannot afford a hard copy, you can always get the eBook.

We have come to the end of this section. Now we will discuss the three different kinds of bipolar disorder—not that I am particularly in favor of labels of disorders because I truly feel all mental disorders have many things in common, including traumatic origins. However, labels can be helpful in making sense of our particular disorder and in helping us recover. They are helpful, but they are not absolute in their own right. It's important to remember that a label is an abstract concept.

Chapter 4 - Three Types of Bipolar Disorder

Broadly speaking, there are three main types of bipolar disorder that can be distinguished by severity, manifestations, and duration of symptoms. While bipolar 1, bipolar 2, and cyclothymia are all characterized by alternating feelings of being high and being low, they differ.

Bipolar 1 Disorder

Bipolar 1 disorder, or bipolar 1, characterized by episodes of mania and deep depression, is the most severe. This is the kind my wife Cheryl suffers from. If not controlled, feelings of being high can escalate into mania. It may begin as a feeling of being high—such is the case with hypomania for bipolar 2, which usually fades after a few days or a week—but it can easily escalate into mania where the person is unable to sleep, becomes irritable, experiences a fast flow of ideas and pressure speech, and tries to communicate everything at once. The result is a word salad of ideas. That is why this more severe bipolar condition has often been mistakenly diagnosed as schizophrenia. To give an example of what may happen, here is what a sufferer wrote to me a while back:

> [Y]ou know, Alfredo, I was writing a poem, and it appeared to me that all of the ideas I ever had, had come to me all at once. All the ideas were flowing out of me and onto the paper. I read it later and I had dozen of pages in front of me. I had been writing poetry the whole day, nonstop. It all made sense at the time but, as I found out later, after being hospitalized, it was nothing but sequences of words that together made little or no sense. But while I was writing it, I felt I had a bestselling poetry book. Ideas escalated so rapidly that my mind switched

off and I cannot remember anything after that. I was told that the mania was so severe that my mind had detached itself from conscious reality. I was hospitalized and with medication came out of the mania.

The question is: Can something be done before the mania kicks in and hospitalization is needed? I would say that in some cases it can. For example, I have worked hard with my wife to avoid mania for many years, and we have succeeded. There is little doubt that in the case of severe bipolar 1, some medication will be needed for many years, and possibly for life; however, it is important to know how much medication (the least amount that will work well); what kind of medication; and what interventions are used, to ensure at least some sleep, to lead a stress-free life, to exercise regularly, to eat well, to have the support of family and friends, and to create a social network. Support is important, but equally important is education. As I mentioned before, sufferers should become their own experts and know as much as possible about their conditions; at the same time, they should also rely on therapists for constant feedback and clarity of judgment.

My wife was hospitalized a number of times, both before and after we got married, but this soon stopped mostly because, as my wife puts it, she now had me to look after her, and she had found love and understanding and someone who would support her, someone like me who also suffered from bipolar 2 and understood her perfectly. This is not one isolated case; many sufferers with bipolar 1 whom I help online have benefitted from my friendship and my ability simply to listen and spend time with them. This tells me there is a strong psychological and mental component to bipolar 1 that has nothing to do with biology, and it is an important aspect of the disorder. Support, and someone who can understand us, are vital to the recovery process.

Recovery for people with bipolar 1 is very possible, but difficult to achieve. What is required is a combination of the right attitude and the right support, especially that of a mental health professional the sufferer has learned to trust; this combination can, in many cases, be combined with the minimum amount of medication that will work. Admittedly, many people with less severe bipolar, such as bipolar 2 and cyclothymia may manage without medication.

More than a Biological Disorder

In America, and to a lesser extent in Australia, many sufferers and mental health professionals firmly believe that bipolar 1 is just a biological disorder that requires medication alone. I have communicated with people who were taking a combination of up to eight different antipsychotics and antidepressants each day. This terrible cocktail of different drugs, with unknown inter-actions, clearly is not conducive to recovery; it stops the functioning of the mind, putting a wrench into the works. While the sufferer may be relieved from the constant pains of the symp-toms and moods, he or she will not be able to recover but will stay in a kind of vegetative state where the mind is so affected by the drugs that the quality of life is reduced drastically and the person will need ever-increasing doses of various medication, even some extra ones, to help with side-effects (Whitfield, L., 2010).

I have often found myself working with sufferers and psychiatrists or psychologists who are friends and who often have advised the person to reduce the amount of medication and begin some sort of psychotherapy or counseling, particularly in cases where PTSD was present. It is widely known, among the better and more educated mental health professionals, that the biopsychosocial model of any mental disorder is the right approach. This means a complete investigation and assessment of biological, psychological, and social factors that affect the person's wellbeing. Unfortunately, even in Australia, there is a tendency among the less skilled mental health professionals to see the problem as purely biological. But here is the problem that is very well known among skilled mental health professionals:

> Conventional psychiatry is plagued by a confusion that lies at the very centre of the conceptual problem of all modern, scientific medicine. Instead of asking why a mental illness occurs, medical researchers try to understand the biological mechanisms through which the illness operates. These mechanisms, rather than true origins, are seen as the causes of the illness. Accordingly,

most current psychiatric treatments are limited to suppressing symptoms with psychoactive drugs. Although they have been successful in doing so, this approach has not helped psychiatrists to understand mental illness any better, nor has it allowed their patients to solve the underlying problems. (R.D. Laing in Capra, 1988)

Helpful Medications

To conclude this brief segment on bipolar 1, if you suffer with it and want to recover, there is always need to attend to psychological (what is in your mind, how you see the problems, and how you respond to life's problem), social (the people around you, are they helpful to you? are they supportive?), and biological in terms of finding the right medication that will help you use the minimum dose possible that will not stump any chance of recovery. Two substances that are very helpful in the treatment of bipolar 1 are lithium and Epilim (sodium valproate). These are effective because they are mood stabilizers as opposed to modern antipsychotics with the more severe side effects. Lithium and Epilim are also older drugs, and their track record has been well documented in contrast to modern antipsychotics that often are not properly tested on humans. However, note that lithium and Epilim have side-effects and some people may be allergic to them.

Frequent blood tests are often required, but the good thing is that these substances stabilize moods and help the person stay calm and focused. They are really good substances and very effective. Psychiatrists are often reluctant to prescribe them because of the constant monitoring required, and because they are invited by pharmaceutical corporations to prescribe new drugs, and as we know, there is a dollar value behind these reasons. But you can ask your psychiatrist to help you try these highly effective substances.

Usually, people on lithium or Epilim take the least amount of medication because these are effective and, with the combination of other natural interventions, very powerful. I say this from experience, not only as a sufferer who is married to a wonderful lady who suffers with bipolar 1 and who was once on lithium and is now on Epilim, but also as someone who is in frequent communication with thousands of sufferers all over the world. The point is that with the mood chemically stabilized, the person can now work on the problem.

Bipolar 2

Bipolar 2 is different from bipolar 1 in that there is no mania. Elevated moods can still cause problems, and deep depression is also present, but the highs never escalate into mania. Still, a person who is experiencing elevated moods in bipolar 2 can suffer with serious problems, and sometimes he or she may also need hospitalization. Most of the symptoms of bipolar 1 are the same except for the absence of mania. Pressure speech, distorted thinking, not needing much sleep, fast flow of ideas, irritability, and an inability to get on well with people when high or depressed will all be present.

These symptoms and moods do not go away in recovery, at least not completely. It is just that the person learns to live well with these to the point that the symptoms and moods become background noise and the person is able to ignore them and continue to live a reasonably good life. Occasionally, these moods and symptoms may regain strength even in the most resilient person, especially if the sufferer experiences traumatic events again, or if for some reason strong memories of past trauma unexpectedly resurface. Even then, the sufferer can experience an episode or two and still get back on the recovery road to continue his or her life.

Cyclothymia

Cyclothymia is the mildest of the three types. It is often called "bipolar light" in America, and it is characterized by frequent alternating moods from highs to lows, sometimes within the same day. This milder form can be troublesome, as the moods and symptoms change rapidly. It is like riding a roller coaster of moods, emotions, and feelings. People with cyclothymia, more so than those with bipolar 1 or 2, may often be driven to excessive alcohol or drug consumption, mostly to cope with the constant changing moods.

It is not easy to put up with this particular disorder because, while many think of it as mild, it is only mild compared to the other two types of bipolar disorder. It is still troublesome in terms of the constant changes, which do affect a person's life quite severely. As is always the case, recovery will not mean that the symptoms go away, but that the person learns to cope with the disorder and is able to live a full life. The idea is that if some people can do it, all people should be able to do it. Just how this could be possible is the aim of this book—to suggest how, regardless of the severity of our condition, we can learn to cope and hop onto the recovery road.

To recapitulate, in terms of elevated moods, hypomania, and mania, there will be some specific symptoms that are universal. These are:

- irritability
- not needing or wanting sleep
- pressure speech
- increased sexual activity
- insensitivity to other people
- feeling one is great or significant or specially chosen
- increased religious/spiritual feelings
- lack of insight
- lack of self-criticism
- spending lots of money
- reduced sense of danger/risk-taking

Depression

Depression is something that nearly one out of three people experience in their lifetimes, to a certain degree (Kessler, 2005). With bipolar disorder, the depression is far greater than that experienced by a normal person. It can be chronic and very deep and can lead to suicidal thoughts.

Symptoms of depression are:

- lack of energy
- change in self-image (feeling ugly and nothing looks right)
- change in sleep patterns (e.g., waking at 3 a.m. and being unable to go back to sleep)
- thoughts of being worthless

- guilt
- wanting to escape one's mind and the constant rumination
- self-centeredness
- feeling emotionally dead
- irritability
- reduced interest in sex
- decreased appetite and interest in food, or comfort eating
- inability to concentrate
- agitation or low energy

When you recover, you will still experience some, or all, of these universal tendencies of the disorder, but you will be able to cope well because, to recover, you will have gained the right skills and knowledge that will help you stay on the road to recovery.

Conclusion

Proper diagnosis is important and, even though labels are guides, not definite disorders, a proper diagnosis can be the difference between recovery or not. In bipolar disorder, it would seem we are confronted with the intensity, concentration, and spread of symptoms, but the characteristics are similar in terms of high and low moods. Many people with bipolar 1 disorder will tell you they have been misdiagnosed in the past as suffering from schizophrenia. This meant they were taking the wrong medication, which worsened, rather than improved, their condition. This has also happened to my wife.

Fortunately, a lot can be done to deal with these substantial problems. At this stage, it is important to look briefly at the biopsychosocial method, according to which a mental disorder must be treated, keeping in mind certain important factors.

No matter how serious your particular bipolar disorder is, there is always hope. Rarely does bipolar comes with psychosis, and only in its most severe form. However, even then there is hope. I will now discuss schizophrenia, a very different disorder from bipolar, simply to show that even in the most severe forms of mental disorder there is hope.

Chapter 5 - The Finnish Open Dialogue Method.

I decided to include the Finnish Open Dialogue Study to argue that there are other ways than our Western method of taking care of people with mental disorders. Some sufferers with bipolar disorder can experience psychosis, a very debilitating condition. But even in such extreme cases, there is hope.

The Open Dialogue is a Finnish approach to treating first-break psychosis, particularly in younger people. It was devised and introduced by a group of family therapists from Tornio, Finland at the Keropudas Hospital in the 1980s. These therapists have been able to change what was once one of the poorest outcomes for schizophrenia in the whole of Europe into a successful way to help sufferers to recover, often permanently. The method has worked time and again, over many years, and many research studies have been conducted with promising outcomes for first break schizophrenia.

The aim is to avoid hospitalization and administration of drugs (early interventions), and to help people recover so they are able to work and get back to their lives. By treating schizophrenia in its earliest stages, they have greatly reduced rates of hospitalization and minimized the need for drugs. Such positive outcomes have captured the attention of many mental health professionals who are dissatisfied with the Western system of treating people with hospitalizations and administration of neuroleptics, which can make things worse in the long run.

The Finnish family therapists work in groups because they see psychosis as a problem that involves relationships. The treatment is based on an *open dialogue* to find the best treatment for the person. The family and friends became a vital part of this treatment, where medication and other problems are discussed openly. The therapists can be a selection from among a psychiatric nurse, a psychiatrist, a psychologist and a family therapist. Mental health experts work in teams of people from various disciplines, which is precisely what makes the treatment powerful. This factor is something we will consider closely as I discuss the film that is freely available online produced by Daniel Mackler who is a therapist, musician, and filmmaker[4]. There is no doubt that this incredibly effective method promotes medication-free recovery, while offering evidence that can be used to critique contemporary psychiatry. Of course, this does not mean that the Open Dialogue method belongs to the Anti-Psychiatry Movement. Indeed the Finnish team does rely on a psychiatrist to lead its team.

One of the biggest critics of this method is Marvin Ross (2013), who states that we need further research to see whether such a method can be used outside Finland. That's ridiculous. There is nothing country-specific in such an approach. It has been successfully used on other issues within the family therapy tradition for many years. Ross then goes on to write that: "a 'filmmaker' produced the video on Open Dialogue." This "filmmaker" was a practicing therapist who decided to become a musician and filmmaker, perhaps due to having lost hope in traditional Western ways of treating people with mental disorders. Ross continues, as Dr. Olsen argues (2014), that when one looks closely at the research, the Open Dialogue method does not really have better results than our current method of early interventions which, in the medical book "*The Merck Manual,* is stated to be at around 30%." In other words, the early interventions of Western societies show a recovery from first episode schizophrenia of 30 percent.

In my experience as an online helper for many people with schizophrenia and their families, there has been very little first episode recovery due to doctors/psychiatrists' interventions. In fact, out of the many hundreds of sufferers, I have not yet heard of one who recovered due to a doctor's intervention. A few days ago, I helped a young man who had experienced his second psychotic episode. Without calling the police, for fear he could end up in jail and, unable to have him committed to our local hospital for lack of beds, I helped him myself with the support of

---

[4] https://www.youtube.com/watch?v=HDVhZHJagfQ

his family, my psychologist friends, and a couple of his friends. He was stabilized after twenty-six hours while we all stayed with him and discussed his problems. We had to help him without medication because his relapse had resulted from discontinuing his medication due to an upset stomach ulcer.

The stories that sufferers with schizophrenia tell me are not about the recovery but the exacerbation of their mental disorders. In fact, people who experience psychosis and are taken to a psychiatric hospital will almost always be restrained, which causes them great anxiety and exacerbates their psychosis. The result is they will be injected with neuroleptics, which, most of the time, will make their condition worse in the long run. Neuroleptics are not a cure.

Dr. Olson (2014) states that statistics show we are now well below the 30 percent recovery mark when it comes to psychosis, and we are gradually losing ground. For example, Wunderink et al. (2013) gives us only 17.6 percent recovery rates for those who had received standard care for a first-time psychotic episode, while Harrow (2007) found that only 5 percent of sufferers recovered with standard care. It is evident now that Ross' idea that the Open Dialogue results are not different from our outcomes in the Western world is based on a false premise.

We do not have 30 percent recovery of first-time psychotic episodes in the Western world simply because our practice is to restrain the person who is experiencing psychosis, take her or him to the hospital, and administer neuroleptic drugs (Mackler, 2014). This experience is very damaging to the psyche of these vulnerable people as psychologist Rufus May[5] argues in his documentary.

Let me add that May had once suffered with schizophrenia. His first-time episode was not one that led to any recovery. By the way, Rufus May uses a similar method to the Open Dialogue to treat people with psychosis, as his documentary clearly shows. And there are other criticisms from Marvin Ross about statistical problems with the research, but I will not go into these because it will mean entering into a debate that is ultimately unhelpful. His critiques have been clearly rendered invalid by Dr. Olsen. The

---

[5] http://www.rufusmay.com/

only critique of Ross that is valid is that we need more research on Open Dialogue to see how it can help the Western world.

I can offer support for this model because I have had to help many people who have suffered with psychotic episodes, including my wife. I can say one of the most beneficial aspects of the Open Dialogue is that it offers support, rather than prejudice. Because the program is a network-based approach, where family members, coworkers, and friends of the client, together with mental health experts, all get together and address the problem, psychosis becomes a social problem. This group support has a tremendous implication for recovery, not the least of which is a watered down, or much reduced, stigma effect. As Rufus May argues (2007):

> Recovery requires other people to believe in and stand by the person. Other people/opportunities play an important part in enabling the person to make this recovery journey

Rufus May and the Recovery Journey

The recovery journey is based on the idea that it is not always the psychosis that is the problem, but rather what people think about the person experiencing the psychosis, their negative judgment, the prejudice, and the stigma. In the Open Dialogue Approach, mental health professionals see the psychosis quite differently from the traditional Western way. As psychologist Rufus May (2007) expresses in his writing, the goal is to see the psychotic experiences as "meaningful events in the context of people's social lives." And this is easily understood when we watch Rufus May's documentary[6] (Regan, 2008).

When I attempt to help someone with psychosis online, the first things I say to the sufferer is that I am very interested in his or her psychotic experiences, and I am not there to judge but to work so that we can try to understand these psychotic events and their important messages. The person may want to talk about the alien spaceship that comes to visit him at night; or how a toy bear talks to her; or how he hears many voices. I accept these experiences as meaningful messages to be understood in the

---

[6] https://www.youtube.com/watch?v=Ffw0pyAjiCw

context of social problems or personal fears and failures. Both the sufferer and I become detectives. I always tell sufferers that we can't worry about the question of whether the psychotic visions are true or not; that is not our immediate concern because they are real in the mind of the sufferer. What is important is that we understand their meaning because, after all, everything we perceive is the creation of our mind, even though we have learned to imagine and create things collectively.

Once the sufferer begins to make sense of his or her psychosis, recovery is not very far, and what also becomes possible is to begin to distinguish the psychosis from everyday reality, the collective reality that we have created. I have seen this happen with my wife and with many friends. Yet they have recovered or are at least able to control their psychosis precisely because they are now aware of the message and purpose of the psychosis. In the great majority of cases, the psychosis is there to protect the sufferers from past traumatic events. But most importantly, it is there to help them express emotions they could not otherwise express. The psychosis serves a vital function, and when this function is understood, in the great majority of cases, the sufferer can move on.

In the film *The Doctor Who Hears Voices* (Regan, 2008) the young doctor, Ruth Fielding, who is experiencing psychosis, says that the psychosis per se is not the main problem; rather, the stigma is, or what others think of the psychosis. The stigma is the real problem that prevents recovery. More specifically, the internalized stigma is the problem: "I am crazy because that is what people think I am."

Rufus May also argues that in recovery, a sufferer learns to cope with his or her difficulties. The vision, psychosis, and related problems may remain, and for some people who learn to cope, these symptoms are no longer a problem but a source of creativity that can enrich a person's life.

What is extremely interesting in this documentary is that Rufus May tells us about his own psychosis. May was invited by Ruth to a conference where a leading psychiatrist (Trevor) was addressing mental health professionals and clients about his new book on schizophrenia. Ruth asked May to tell Trevor his ideas were misguided and that the recovery concept was missing from his book. May then tells Trevor that he does not listen to his patients and he is misguided by his training, by his profession. At this point, Trevor becomes quite upset, asking May how he knows that he does not listen to his patients? May replies that he knows because many years ago he was one of his patients, although he is now a professional psychologist.

In fact, May was suffering from psychosis at age eighteen and was taken away, without his consent, to a psychiatric hospital where he was injected and subjected to a very uncaring and unsympathetic medical system of treating people with schizophrenia, which usually does more harm than good. Detained in an intimidating ward, May was told that he would never recover and that he would have to be on medication for the rest of his life. As we learn, May discontinued his medication once out of the hospital, and went on to become a clinical psychologist.

May's documentary is worth watching because it shows that people with psychosis can recover, sometimes even without medication, as was the case for May and Ruth. It can also be used to support the principles of the Open Dialogue Approach.

The Open Dialogue Approach

Ole Larsen, a Danish psychiatrist, who has used the Open Dialogue approach in various areas of Denmark, states that the approach is not just a way of thinking, but a practical method, a way in which psychiatry has been organized within the social sector in Finland. The method has developed over a number of years using "The Need Adapted Treatment" for psychosis. The idea was that psychotherapy could be used with people who suffered with psychosis. It supported sufferers with safe places to live and offered them jobs. The results were so positive that the Open Dialogue Approach has dominated the West Lappland region of Finland for some years.

Although for a while the Open Dialogue method was forgotten, in West Lappland it continues to develop, and many therapists from all over the world have become puzzled by this method, although it makes a lot of sense to people who have experienced psychosis, including therapists like Rufus May and Mary Olsen.

The network meeting that takes place, involving family, coworkers, and friends of the client, and which is an essential part of the Open Dialogue approach, is based on the work of Tom Anderson from Tromso, Norway, and is called the "reflecting processes." Anderson's central philosophy is that in any discussion, we have an inner and outer dialogue and the need to sit and listen without needing to answer.

One important thing about the Open Dialogue approach is that a lot of things we often consider to be trivial are all so important. For example, one of the policies of the Finnish professionals who use this method is to answer the phone immediately, no matter what one is doing.

In the film, we notice that while mental health professionals are filmed, they interrupt the conversation to answer the phone. This is because picking up the phone can make the difference between saving a life or not, and their policy is that no matter what they are doing, someone needs to answer that phone. The support starts from the moment the phone rings. This responsiveness is a far cry from what happens here in Australia where sufferers have to wait long periods of time before they get any treatment. Sometimes, it is quicker for them to end up in jail than it is to get help, given that often their first intervention is a call to the police, who are often inexperienced in interacting with people who are experiencing psychosis.

Psychosis and Open Dialogue

What happens when someone experiencing psychosis, or a family member, partner, or friend, rings up for help?

Nurse Pahivi Vathola:

> When we pick up the phone and someone needs us to help, we don't say to them that we are going to arrange things within two weeks. We arrange things immediately.
>
> When the phone rings, you pick it up and you are responsible from then on. It's a question of being available to people and helping the population...you never know what the phone call is about. It could be a mother worried about her son having developed a psychotic experience and then I have to start organizing things immediately so that we can help promptly before something goes wrong.

We aim at the democratic system where people can have a say about their own treatment and discuss this with the group. To help this process, mental health professionals try to discuss the problems with the client as equal human beings.

We don't claim to know everything. We don't go there and after one hour tell the family what is wrong with the client. It takes time to recognize the problems and to think of possible solutions through open dialogue.

We like the idea of listening to people and together creating something that can help them as a group team effort. We don't worry so much about labels but treating the person as a unique individual who needs a particular kind of support and help and who can participate to their recovery if they wish. The place where we receive calls can be just a tiny room with a phone, computer, and printer/fax.

We just organize things from a room because we don't want people to come to hospital, we don't have many beds available, and our aim is to treat the person in their social settings, often going to their places or organizing things in other venues. The aim is to organize a place where we can meet and begin the dialogue. If hospitalization is absolutely necessary, then we have that, but our aim is to avoid hospitalizations and administration of potent drugs.

Therapist and filmmaker Mackler tells the journalist that the Open Dialogue approach is famous. He heard of it in the United States. He says:

I've heard of it in conferences in Scandinavia, I've heard of it from friends in England, but mostly by reading the work and research of psychologist Jaakko Seikkula...

Indeed, the Finnish team of therapists that first adopted the Open Dialogue method consisted of Jaakko Seikkula, Brigitta Alakare, and Markku Sutela, with support from nurses and other staff members. This team operated at the Keropudas Hospital in Tornio, back in 1980.

For Professor Jaakko Seikkula, who works at the University of Jyväskylä, the Open Dialogue approach works well, but it was difficult to develop because the initial team made lots of mistakes in the program's early stages. Nevertheless, Mackler argues, the West Lappland of Finland have the best results for the treatment of first-break psychosis in the entire world. The evidence from over thirty years of treating people in Finland shows that people recover there while they do not in the rest of the world. That is what is so interesting to many therapists. In my opinion, we have evidence here that, in the near future, a universal method of treatment could be devised because we have enough knowledge and experience to do so. We also have enough supporting evidence to convince us this is the way to the future—to treat the person first with all of his or her social and psychological problems and only as a last resort to turn to medication or the biological problems.

Treatment as Intervention

According to Jaakko Seikkula, getting the family, friends of the client, and the therapists, nurses, and other staff all in one room is a way to use the meeting as an intervention to introduce possible change within the family. As the Seikkula clarifies, we are still the therapists and we have to have aims, make the decisions, and follow a logical sequence of interventions, but we do this in a democratic way in discussion with the client and his or her family and friends. Both the family and client, in doing so, become active agents of the treatment process.

The client needs to be there from the very beginning as treatment is discussed. Treatment may consist of administration of some medication, discussion of problems troubling the client, what the family can do to accommodate the client's needs, and how the client can change, if required, to get the best support from his or her family. The same applies in the workplace. In other words, psychosis is mostly seen as a social problem, not just an internal problem of the mind to be treated biochemically.

Clearly, where we are going wrong in the Western world is we are so busy giving diagnosis, prescribing medication, labeling people, and doing all of these biomedical procedures that we often forget what is important: that people with psychosis, no matter how serious, can recover. It has happened many times.

What prevents people from recovery is mostly our ideology that people with psychosis are incurable and permanently damaged.

This way of looking at the problem is ideal for those who see it from a biomedical perspective and want to treat the problem by medicating it. But, as we know, medication is not a complete treatment; at best, it is useful in the initial stages, but sooner or later, as I have argued previously, the client or sufferer needs to work toward recovery. In addition, many people recover without medication.

This way of intervening and acting is very uncommon in the Western world. However, it is the way to the future treatment of mental disorders. This book can be considered a contribution to this future, and hopefully, it will help readers achieve change. It does not offer a biomedical way of doing things but more of a psychosocial method, with the inclusion of some biomedical intervention when needed. In short, this method is biopsychosocial.

A last important thought is that positive change toward recovery happens as a consequence of dialogue. I am sure many therapists would agree with me when I say that once we help the person from a person-centered perspective, not an exclusively medical one, it is likely we'll get good results because we are engaging with the person in a discussion of how to solve problems, which are not entirely biological but that have to do with the psychological wellbeing of the person and his or her environment. This is not only logical but an inconvenient truth for the Western world.

Concluding Thoughts

In conclusion, it can be said that actors develop a special empathy by putting themselves in their characters' shoes. Characters always have stories, personalities, and lots of reasons for developing as they have. Like a snowflake in the wind, which is shaped by currents and strong winds, so too personality is shaped by life experiences and our environment. It may seem impossible to us, but, in reality, it is not impossible to change the story of our life. Indeed, to recover, it is sometimes necessary to change one's life or make substantial changes that will make it possible for us to recover. For example, if you have a major problem at home, it is unlikely recovery will be possible until you eliminate the problem.

Consider a woman who lives with a violent partner. Troubled by constant domestic violence, she will be traumatized every day and the trauma will increase every day. In this situation, recovery will be absolutely impossible. She will either need to make sure her partner seeks help or she will need to distance herself and leave her partner for good. Only then will she be able to recover. What happens in your environment is important, so if you want to recover, you have to ensure you do not have overwhelming problems that will prevent you from recovering. Of course, if you have a good therapist, he will tell you this and help you. For people with bipolar disorder, a therapist is necessary.

By developing empathy, we make progress toward the elimination of stigma and prejudice in mental health, which are major sources of suicidal ideation and mental ill health. The acting profession can teach us how to develop empathy and how to learn about people by putting ourselves in their shoes. We should look at this inquiry closely so we can truly help people with mental disorders in a much more efficient, healthier, and more hopeful manner.

I remember a time when I was homeless, with not a cent in my pocket, living in my car outside a mental health hospital. You can read all about it in my book *Alfredo's Journey: An Artist's Creative Life with Bipolar Disorder*. I was admitted into the hospital not because I was mad but because I was homeless and depressed. I was helped there, and it was there that I first begun to practice method acting to get better. Of course, in those days I had no knowledge of method acting, but the actions I took were very similar to method acting: I imagined I was happy, that for the first time I could abandon my old depressed self and let people help me. I imagined I could restore my life into something normal and that I could become a good person, a hard worker, someone others could respect no matter what. I did it and my life slowly changed. My wife has a similar story that you can also read it in my book. Returning to a normal life can be done.

Chapter 6 - The Biopsychosocial Model of Mental Health

As will be seen from the kind of biopsychosocial model of mind I briefly outline in this chapter, science is more than a way of studying phenomena in the laboratory, where naïve materialism relies on the idea that in order to understand a given phenomenon, it needs to be broken down into smaller parts. The idea is that once studied, the small parts can be reassembled later on to understand the whole. This is highly inadequate for the biopsychosocial model of mind. To give an example, scientists are trying to explain consciousness in terms of deconstructing it into a series of parts, much like a machine to be disassembled and reassembled. They are convinced that consciousness arises from brain function (see professor Steven Pinker) and they dismiss the extensive research on past lives and near-death experiences that provide evidence that consciousness can continue to exist outside of the body. For many years, scientists have conducted research on past lives, and the bulk of their research cannot be dismissed. (See the research of Dr. Ian Stevenson and Jim Tucker.)

The kind of naïve materialism I am speaking of has entered many academic institutions and is a barrier to real progress, despite the fact that following the ideas of Samuel and his Multimodal Framework, it is pretty clear that a new paradigm of mind is emerging. It has been emerging for quite a few years now, and more than likely, it will begin to crystallize soon. We are beginning to know how the brain works, particularly because of our ability, through science, to look at fMRI brain scans and other methods where we can see electro-chemical activities that drive behavior.

Yet the more we understand about the brain, the more elusive consciousness becomes. Just what is it that makes me conscious that I am alive, in the world today, and able to feel what is happening to and around me, making me aware of my presence on Earth? Some would say it is an effect of the brain that gives us the illusion of consciousness. What a stupid way to look at this phenomenon. Fortunately for me and my brain and mind, there is far too much evidence of the afterlife and existence outside of the body that cannot be dismissed; only ignorant people can dismiss this today as nonsense. What is important to emphasize now, which I will explore in the following chapter, is that in psychology today, there are two distinct groups of psychologists: those like Howard Gardner who believe that psychology is above all an art, an art that needs to be supported by science; and those like Susan Blackmore who believe that psychology is primarily a science.

For the scientific psychologists, any notion of the fictional self (because we all use fiction to make sense of our lives; we create stories and become the central characters in the stories) should be banished to make room for the neuron-centered, scientific psychology. For the artistic psychologists, the fictional self is the firm foundation from which the person can be studied and helped by focusing on what makes us human that cannot be studied scientifically. What makes us human is our will, our consciousness, our empathy, our ability to engage in emotions, and our need for friendship and cooperation. These human tendencies can be researched scientifically, but they are not scientific and belong to the art realm of psychology used by therapists.

Psychology and Art

When I say art in psychology, I am referring to the use of creativity, art, dialogue, and friendship in psychology. These are the elements I use each day to help people. In fact, I do not use science at all in my voluntary effort to help people find a better way to exist. I believe countries that embrace this new emerging paradigm, based on the union of science, art, and spirituality, will be able to move forward, while those that do not will be left behind. By spirituality, I mean all the phenomena in the world that we cannot explain, such as consciousness. I can see how Australia is being left behind by some other countries that are now beginning to embrace a more inclusive science. Interestingly, a good friend, an academic, Bill Bottomley, once told me that explaining consciousness is like chewing one's teeth. But if we must guard against naïve materialism, we must also guard against naïve idealism. Naïve idealism proposes that it is possible for all people to see auras, to feel the presence of spirits, and to have visions of the future. Clearly, we must be cautious; while paranormal phenomena are possible, there are also many unscrupulous people who will prey on our desire to experience such phenomena.

We must be open-minded but never naïve; naïve materialism and naïve idealism are both highly problematic. We must guard against both. I will argue that science, seen as a paradigm, is very limited because of the corruption and lack of transparency found at many levels of its practice and application. Bogus research, which serves the interest of powerful corporations and materialists, who use science for their own ends, driven by ideology that is akin to dogma, impacts people's hope that science will be an independent, transparent, and honest method of studying life for the improvement of the human condition, and not for financial gains and the increased power of a few. If they haven't noticed by now, untrustworthy people should know that their game is being exposed. At another level, reducing all religions to dogma is also problematic because, as scientist Susan Greenfield states, science and religion can sometimes work together.

Meditation and Mindfulness

For example, if we consider Buddhism to be a non-theistic religion, then the use of meditation and mindfulness in psychology could do well with a little help from this religion. As Professor Samuel argues, there are problems with the way in which the Western world has incorporated mindfulness into its practice: one problem is that it has largely dismissed the concept of Non-Self, one of the main concepts of mindful activities; and the science of mindfulness could also benefit from a closer investigation of the Subtle Body concept, which roughly corresponds to the work of Carl Jung and Sigmund Freud on the unconscious, dreams, sexual drives, the ego, archetypes, and so on—things that belong more to the artistic side of psychology. It is a pity that we have largely dismissed the work of Sigmund Freud and Carl Jung in psychology. Although many of their theories were problematic, and some have even been discredited, their direction was an important one we should not abandon. They provided an understanding for how science and spirituality could work well together. Indeed, I use aspects of Buddhism to help people.

The concept of non-self is useful in helping people to distance themselves from the obsessive rumination and constant inner turmoil they constantly find themselves in. Part of my effort to help is to explain to people that they can put aside the idea of a self by taking deep breaths and imagining that they are part of a greater whole, that they are connected to the universe, and that they are an important part of the creation. This also goes well with the effort of the actor who has to distance him- or herself from the self to assume a new personality and character. This works well for me, although it takes considerable effort to help someone begin to practice this kind of therapeutic meditation in order to distance oneself from the self. But it works in most cases, and as people learn to distance themselves from their selves, the will often takes over—the will to get better, to see things differently, to try new things, to trust. Give people an adequate mental environment, and they will help themselves. I learned this from Buddhism, not from science.

Toward a Spiritual Science

Another concern is to look at the heated debate of psychology as a science versus the claim that it isn't. I would like to make it perfectly clear that this book proposes that the only way forward, for psychology, is to become a "spiritual science," but a spiritual science that has nothing to do with scientology. I know the term could upset some psychologists and academics, but the fact is that as long as psychology is confronted by research on past lives, investigations into consciousness, near-death experiences, and similar unresolved dilemmas that fit well into the spiritual realm, at least for now, it makes good sense to study these phenomena in a responsible manner.

This means we must admit such phenomena exist, because we cannot dismiss the research findings, and attempt to use the scientific method to understand such phenomena rather than discard it as mumbo jumbo, something we can no longer afford to do. Is psychology a science? Absolutely, but it is also concerned with that part of humanity that cannot be explained scientifically. Hence, it is a spiritual science and, I would add, it is much superior to hard science because it is aware of the spiritual and unexplainable aspects of life.

It is important for me now to emphasize that psychology has taken a turn for the worse. Currently, it is basing its efforts on the scientific method, or more precisely, the scientific reductionism that leads to naïve materialism. It is a fact that we need a lot more focus on the person, and it is also a fact, as Gardner argues, that literature and history are of the outmost importance for psychology because they provide information about aspects of humanity that are not quantifiable in naïve materialistic terms, and yet are so very important for an understanding of how humans tick, what drives us, and what motivates us. Here we find a great dilemma because, as someone who helps many sufferers online and as a person who has many psychologists and psychiatrists as friends, I can say that science is of little use in therapy.

Do therapists use science? No, they do not use science. They may get some information from science, occasionally, and perhaps use the recommendations in their daily practices, but as an online helper for sufferers, I can say that I get my information not from science but from my understanding of Buddhism; and I can also say that I am much more effective in helping people psychologically than many of my friends who are psychologists or psychiatrists. And I like to remind people that I do this work as a volunteer so that, even if I am not qualified as a therapist, I can still help people who suffer, as I have in the past.

How many therapists use statistics? How many need biology and chemistry? I have asked a few psychologists and psychiatrists these questions and they all tell me they haven't used statistics in years, and they have forgotten most things about biology and chemistry. They do not use science in this way. I am not implying that science is not important for psychology, because I believe it is; what I am implying is that we should spend a lot more time teaching future psychologists about the person (person-centered practices, see Carl Rogers), and the literature of humanity, philosophy, and history. It is here that, ironically, scientific research tells us person-centered practices are highly successful in helping people. Why is this? Humans are storied beings. This means we make sense of our life by creating stories in our mind and becoming central characters of our life story. We follow a fixed script in which we know who we are in relation to other people such as friends, coworkers, and family members. If this is true, and it is, then an actor should be able to change the script and act accordingly.

Changing the Script

Sometimes the life script of people changes by necessity, because of dramatic life events such as the loss of a job and related identity, or the loss of a partner due to death. These are dramatic events that create script changes and are very traumatic. In order to study these events and help people, a therapist can rely on research, and evidence-based practices, but the effort to help is mostly creative and belongs to the realm of art. I believe there is not focus on creativity and art in the undergraduate psychology courses, which may well affect the outcome of undergraduate studies. For example, I can say with confidence that undergraduate studies based on scientific reductionism are doing some damage: psychologists who come out at the end of the four years' honors course, and who are going to become therapists, are lacking in the area of person-centered studies. I say this because I know many psychologists, some of whom I help daily, who lack understanding of the practical aspects of mental disorders and how they are shaped by life events, experience, and the environment. It is important to understand that when I speak of science, I don't mean the kind of reductionism that is part of the hardcore sciences.

For the study of human beings, we need a much broader science that is aware of the fact that, as Thomas Khun (1963) argued, scientific paradigms have a tendency to be replaced by new ones and scientific facts are often proven false as new under-standings of life are introduced. For example, we went from the universe of Newton and Galileo of the seventeenth century, to the universe of Einstein, Schrödinger, and Heisenberg in the nineteenth century when quantum theory revolutionized the way we understand particles and the universe.

I confidently speculate that the next step is consciousness. I believe that consciousness studies will possibly replace the quantum understanding of life. No doubt, they will also be replaced by another paradigm. For example, we once believed the Earth was flat till the day when science proved to us it is spherical. Science is only a method, a valuable method that helps us understand the "phenomenon of the day," but it is not something that can lead us to absolute truth as certain hardcore scientists would have us believe. I cannot emphasize this more! We need a science that can deal with the unexplainable, and as such, is open to the fact that it cannot explain everything, but that it still needs to include the phenomena as a valuable study, not dismiss it as hard core scientists do: "We cannot understand something; therefore, it is not part of science." Sweeping it under the carpet is clearly not the way to go for psychology. If we cannot understand something, the idea is to study it until we understand it better. Qualitative methods can always be used to compare data or understand phenomena.

The Study of Human Beings

Part of the biopsychosocial method is to propose an adequate science for the study of human beings. From this book, I hope you will become aware of the many problems that affect society from the perspective of someone who understands quite well both the working class and middle class academics. In this sense, I have tried to establish an intellectual bridge where the concern of the poor people, people who are often silenced by their inability to express themselves, or by fear or for other reasons, can be taken right to the doorstep of the middle and upper classes.

That is why I comfortably say to governments that it is time to wake up and stop playing political games; it is time to look at the long-term impact of your policies, not the short-term one; and it is time to become responsible people rather than showing the wisdom of a two-year-old toddler. We need mature politicians who can guide the country. We need corporations that become responsible because they realize they play a crucial role in society. It is time to stop the greed and corruption and try to help the world, a world that is in a state of chaos and fast deteriorating.

These are some of the many concerns of the biopsychosocial model, a model that, in order to work for us properly, needs transparency, honesty, and people's will to create a better, more just world. I think most people desire this, and as time goes by, we realize something needs to be done about stupid governments and corrupt corporations. It is clear now that I cannot offer a polished and perfectly specific biopsychosocial model. That would be silly. I can only point toward our future direction, the road less travelled, that could potentially take us to the realization of a biopsychosocial model for the creation of better policies, a better understanding of the mind, and a better future. If I can point toward this, then I will achieve something; no matter how small this effort may be, it is a step in the right direction. For people with mental disorders, it is important to attend to environmental, social, and psychological factors, not just biological ones. The mistake many first world countries are making is to focus on biology alone when it is not, by itself, going to help people recover.

Conclusion

I hope that by reading this book, you will have come to understand that humans are *storied* beings. That means we understand our lives in terms of the stories we tell ourselves, our friends, our families, and other people. Our mental activity is created by the mind, but the abstract stories we construct and those that constantly emerge from our fantasies do have a real impact on our lives.

Taking medication alone is not enough. We need to analyze our life story, try to find problems, and see whether we can somehow solve them or at least reduce them so we can recover. In this sense, although hardcore psychiatrists, who rely on a biological explanation of mental disorder, seeing it as an illness, will want to banish any notion of stories or fiction from treatment, stories and fiction are important. That is why mental health professionals who pay attention to stories and fiction are the best. They will strongly believe in the biopsychosocial model of treatment.

As you have probably found out at this point, there is need to do a lot of work in order to get on the road to recovery. If you are not already on the road to recovery, you can get on it. We all can. Start studying your life story, and see whether you can change the script so you can get on the road to recovery.

Good luck, and please, work on the tools offered in this book so you can achieve better mental health. This book was written mostly with the intention to help people like my wife and me.

Thank you for reading.

Appendix: Therapeutic Readings

Desiderata

We all have a higher self inside of us, a self that instinctively knows how to help us help ourselves. It is important to get in touch with this higher self and learn how to be in harmony with the energy of the Universe. Max Ehermann wrote the Desiderata letter in 1927 and it has become more popular each year. It is helpful to read this letter over and over to understand fully its important message:

~ ~ ~

Go placidly amid the noise and the haste, and remember what peace there may be in silence.

As far as possible, without surrender, be on good terms with all persons. Speak your truth quietly and clearly; and listen to others, even to the dull and the ignorant; they too have their story. Avoid loud and aggressive persons; they are vexatious to the spirit.

If you compare yourself with others, you may become vain or bitter, for always there will be greater and lesser persons than yourself. Enjoy your achievements as well as your plans. Keep interested in your own career, however humble; it is a real possession in the changing fortunes of time.

Exercise caution in your business affairs, for the world is full of trickery. But let this not blind you to what virtue there is; many persons strive for high ideals, and everywhere life is full of heroism. Be yourself. Especially do not feign affection. Neither be cynical about love, for in the face of all aridity and disenchantment, it is as perennial as the grass.

Take kindly the counsel of the years, gracefully surrendering the things of youth. Nurture strength of spirit to shield you in sudden misfortune. But do not distress yourself with dark imaginings. Many fears are born of fatigue and loneliness.

Beyond a wholesome discipline, be gentle with yourself. You are a child of the universe no less than the trees and the stars; you have a right to be here. And whether or not it is clear to you, no doubt the universe is unfolding as it should.

Therefore be at peace with God, whatever you conceive Him to be. And whatever your labors and aspirations, in the noisy confusion of life, keep peace in your soul.

With all its sham, drudgery, and broken dreams, it is still a beautiful world. Be cheerful. Strive to be happy.

The Cracked Pot

Therapeutic writing can be very healing and helpful to those who suffer with bipolar disorder. Look for and collect such writings. Read them from time to time; they will be very helpful in ways you cannot even imagine.

~ ~ ~

A water bearer in India had two large pots. Each hung on each end of a pole, which he carried across his neck. One of the pots had a crack in it, and while the other pot was perfect and always delivered a full portion of water at the end of the long walk from the stream to the master's house, the cracked pot arrived only half full.

For a full two years this went on daily, with the bearer delivering only one and a half pots full of water in his master's house. Of course, the perfect pot was proud of its accomplishments, perfect for the end for which it was made. But the poor cracked pot was ashamed of its own imperfection, and miserable that it was able to accomplish only half of what it had been made to do.

After two years of what it perceived to be a bitter failure, it spoke to the water bearer one day by the stream. "I am ashamed of myself, and I want to apologise to you. "Why?" asked the bearer. "What are you ashamed of?" "I have been able, for these past two years, to deliver only half my load because this crack in my side causes water to leak out all the way back to your master's house. Because of my flaws, you have to do all of this work, and you don't get full value from your efforts," the pot said.

The water bearer felt sorry for the old cracked pot, and in his compassion he said, "As we return to the master's house, I want you to notice the beautiful flowers along the path." Indeed, as they went up the hill, the old cracked pot took notice of the sun warming the beautiful wild flowers on the side of the path, and this cheered it somewhat. But at the end of the trail, it still felt bad because it had leaked out half its load, and so again it apologized to the bearer for its failure.

The bearer said to the pot, "Did you notice that there were flowers only on your side of your path, but not on the other pot's side? That's because I have always known about your flaw, and I took advantage of it. I planted flower seeds on your side of the path, and every day while we walk back from the stream, you've watered them. For two years I have been able to pick these beautiful flowers to decorate my master's table. Without you being just the way you are, he would not have this beauty to grace his house."

References

Beers, M. (2015). *The Merck manual of diagnosis and therapy* (18th ed.) (R. S. Porter & T. V. Jones, Eds.). Whitehouse Station, NJ: Merck Sharp & Dohme Cor.

Capra, F. (1989). *Uncommon wisdom: Conversations with remarkable people.* Flamingo: Hammersmith, London.

Clay, S. (1990) in Onken, S. J., Craig, C. M., Ridgway, P., Ralph, R. O., & Cook, J. A. (2007). An analysis of the definitions and elements of recovery: A review of the literature. *Psychiatric Rehabilitation Journal* 31 (1): 9-22.

Clay, S. (1997). *Empowerment and recovery*, [online]. Available: http://home.earthlink.net/~sallyclay/Z.text/empowerment.html [accessed: 20.03.17]

Corry, A., Tubridy, A. (2001). *Going mad? Understanding Mental Illness.* Newleaf: Dublin.

Doidge, N. (2007). *The brain that changes itself: Stories of personal triumph from the frontiers of brain science.* New York: Viking.

Felitti, V. J. et. al (1998) Relationship of Childhood Abuse and Household Dysfunction to Many of the Leading Causes of Death in Adults. *American Journal of Preventive Medicine.* Vol. 14: 245–25.

Harris, Thomas A. (1973). *I'm OK—You're OK.* Pan Books, London, Sydney, Auckland.

Kessler, R. C., Berglund, P., Demler, O., Walters, E. E., & Jin, R. (2005). Lifetime Prevalence and Age-of-Onset Distributions of DSM-IV Disorders in the National Comorbidity Survey Replication. *Archives of General Psychiatry* 62 (6): 593-602.

Kaminski, Battaglia, M. (2002) *Aa hermeneutic historical study of Kazimierz Dabrowski and his theory of positive disintegration.* Falls Church, Virginia. Retrieved from https://theses.lib.vt.edu/theses/available/etd-04082002-204054/unrestricted/Dissertation.pdf

Kuhn, T. S. (1963). *The structure of scientific revolutions. Chicago: University* of Chicago Press.

Mackler, D. (Director). (2014). Open Dialogue: an alternative Finnish approach to healing psychosis [Motion picture]. Retrieved from https://www.youtube.com/watch?v=HDVhZHJagfQ.

May, R. (2006). *Understanding psychotic experiences.* Retrieved from https://www.mentalhealthforum.net/forum/thread3348.html

McGruder, J. (2001). Life Experience Is Not a Disease or Why Medicializing Madness Is Counterproductive to Recovery. *Occupational Therapy in Mental Health, 17, 59-80.*

Olson, M. (2014). The Promise of Open Dialogue. Retrieved November 21, 2017, from https://www.madinamerica.com/2014/01/promise-open-dialogue-response-marvin-ross

O'Neill, L. (2015). Demands of acting hurting performers' mental health. Retrieved November 19, 2017, from https://sydney.edu.au/news-opinion/news/2015/09/14/demands-of-acting-hurting-performers--mental-health.htm

Pearson,C., Mann, S., Zotti, A., (2016) *Art therapy and the creative process: A practical approach.* Loving Healing Press, Ann Arbor.

Regan L. (Director), (2008). *The Doctor who hears voices.* [Motion picture]. UK: Kudos Film and Television. Retrieved from https://www.youtube.com/watch?v=Ffw0pyAjiCw

Reznik, O. (2011). *The secrets of medical decision making: How to avoid becoming a victim of the health care machine* (Kindle Edition), Loving Healing Press.

Shannon, C., Douse, K., McCusker, C., Feeney, L., Barrett, S., & Mulholland, C. (2011). The Association Between

Childhood Trauma and Memory Functioning in Schizophrenia. *Schizophrenia Bulletin, 37*(3), 531–537. http://doi.org/10.1093/schbul/sbp096

Spaniol, L., Wewiorski, N., Gagne, C. Anthony, W.A., (2002) The process of recovery from schizophrenia. *International Review of Psychiatry*, 14(4), 327-336.

Spaniol, L., Gagne, C., & Koehler, M. (1999). Recovery from serious mental illness: What it is and how to support people in their recovery. In R. P. Marinelli & A. E. Dell Orto (Eds.), *The psychological and social impact of disability* (4th ed.). New York: Springer Publishing.

Whitfield, L. (2010) Psychiatric Drugs as Agents of Trauma Excerpted from: *The International Journal of Risk Factorf & Safety in Medicine* 22 (2010) 195-207 DOI 10.3233/185-2010-0508

Whittaker, R. (2016). The Case Against Antipsychotics: A Review of Their Long-term Effects. Retrieved from http://www.madinamerica.com/wp-content/uploads/2016/07/The-Case-Against-Antipsychotics.pdf

Zotti, A. (2014). *Alfredo's Journey: An Artist's Creative Life with Bipolar Disorder*. Loving Healing Press, Ann Arbor.

About the Author

Alfredo Zotti is the son of the late Luciano Zotti (https://it.wikipedia.org/wiki/Luciano_Zotti), Italian composer, orchestra conductor, and musical director, and his wife, Cristina Zotti.

Alfredo, his parents, and brother Giovanni migrated to Sydney, Australia in 1974. At first, life was difficult because the family worked in a wood factory for little pay. As time went on, Luciano began to work as a musician and music teacher and life slowly improved for him and his family.

In 1981, after many traumatic events, Alfredo began his lifelong challenge of living with bipolar disorder. He quickly hit rock bottom, spending time as a homeless person and turning to street drugs and alcohol to medicate his symptoms. But life improved after hospitalization and careful outpatient monitoring.

Alfredo married Cheryl MacDonald, who also suffers with bipolar disorder, and he was able to enrol in a university course. He gained an honours degree in sociology and anthropology. He went on to study clinical psychology at the University of Newcastle, but he did not complete his degree because he felt that academia had taken the wrong path in the prevention and cure of mental illnesses. He completed some courses at first, second, and third year level, with distinction and high distinction. Alfredo also studied piano and was able to gain the 8th year piano grade.

Today, Alfredo is the full-time caregiver for his wife, who suffers from a number of disabilities. He also regularly raises funds for his local hospital, Gosford Hospital, by organizing fundraiser nights where he plays with other musicians. So far, he has helped to raise thousands of dollars. The money goes toward the needs of the hospital's patients with mental disorders. Alfredo also writes an online journal, *The Anti Stigma*

Crusaders, which he uploads regularly at two or three month intervals.

Alfredo also provides support for online sufferers and uses his art to help people. While he is not a qualified music therapist, he does use music and art to help people online. Some mental health professionals often consult him for his lived experience and knowledge of psychology and music. He has written three books, including this one, two published and one that is free online. He also contributes by giving talks in universities about his experience with bipolar disorder.

Index

More than a just a journey, Alfredo gives us a blueprint for humane treatment of mental illness

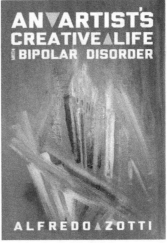

In 1981, twenty-three-year-old Alfredo Zotti began his lifelong challenge of living with Bipolar 2 Disorder. He quickly hit rock bottom, spending time as a homeless person and turning to street drugs and alcohol to medicate his symptoms. After hospitalization and careful out-patient monitoring, he became a successful musician and completed university. In 2004, he started to mentor sufferers of mental illness, and together, they developed an online journal. Alfredo now sees mental illness from a new perspective, not of disadvantages but advantages. In his words: "Having a mental illness can be a blessing if we work on ourselves."

In this memoir and critique of mental illness, the reader will learn:
- How empathic listening and being with someone can help calm that person's symptoms
- The power of singing to create a safe space in a community
- Why spirituality can be a key component in the healing process
- The connections between mental illness, artistic expression, and people who think differently
- The impact of childhood trauma on our psyche and its role in mental illness
- The dangers of antipsychotics and antidepressants
- The amazing connection between heart and brain and how we can cultivate it
- The challenges of love and marriage between partners with Bipolar Disorder

ISBN 978-1-61599-224-9
From Modern History Press

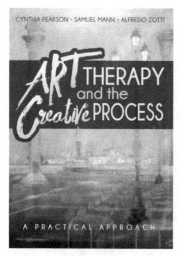

International voices from across the globe come together in *Art Therapy and the Creative Process* to share their perspectives on art, the artist's process, and how art has been therapeutic for them.

In the first section, the three primary contributors—Alfredo Zotti, Samuel Mann, and Cynthia Pearson—create a triple commentary on a piece of art. Zotti paints a picture, Mann analyzes it, and Pearson writes a poem to complement it. In later sections, various artists share why they write, paint, play music, or take photographs, including what their individual mediums mean to them, what they may mean to others, why they have chosen various art forms, how art allows them an opportunity to escape from the world, and how it can also help them heal.

Artists will find kindred spirits in these pages. Lovers of literature, music, and art in all its forms will gain insight into artists' souls, how they view the world a little differently, and why. *Art Therapy and the Creative Process* gives art a purpose beyond what most of us usually think of it having—that art is a way to keep us all sane in a maddening world, and it gives us the opportunity to create something to heal that same world that wounds us.

"This book is a beautiful piece of work and all concerned should be very proud. The human dimension is enhanced through art and expressive approaches should be a much stronger part of mental health care."
— Professor Patrick McGorry, AO MD PhD, Executive Director, OYH Research Centre, University of Melbourne

ISBN 978-1-61599-296-6
From Loving Healing Press